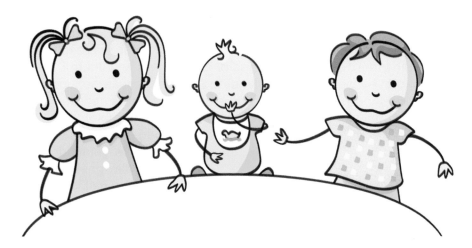

Yummy Yum For Everyone

Denise McCabe

The purpose of this book is to share recipes of a Mom that leaves out the most common food allergens. This book does not, however, constitute professional advice regarding any child or individual's food allergies or nutrition nor is it meant to imply that these recipes are safe for every child. Please consult your pediatric allergist to discuss how foods in this book may have an affect on your child. Additionally this book does not intend to suggest that every food in here is suitable for every baby, toddler or child. It is up to the parents discretion to determine which foods are suitable for their children at their given ages, as well as to cut food into appropriate sizes.

This book is dedicated to Owen who teaches me
the wonders of being a Mom each day and to
all babies and children with food allergies
and their parents who ask for better.

Special thanks to my husband John
who never doubted this would happen
and to the following friends and their children:
Rebecca MacLachlan, Tim MacLachlan,
Gannon MacLachlan, Ainsley MacLachlan,
Alicea Charamut Gerwien, Sean Gerwien,
Isabelle Guinard Kelly and Nina Xixis.

Notes

Contents

Contents (Continued)

Yummy Yum Desserts

When you have lemons, MAKE LEMONADE...

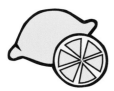 I once worked in a full time job and ate the way most busy people do – without thought and mostly out of a box or through takeout. When my son Owen started to exhibit signs of allergy to dairy at 3 months of age, our world began to change. What I didn't know then was it would be for the better, as it prompted our family to play an active role in what we were eating. In many ways Owen started to uncover the hidden truths about the world of fast paced eating in which we all live. He could not tolerate foods with pesticides or processed foods with long lists of ingredients (he was bound to react to one of them). I began to see new meaning in living AND EATING simply. This began my search to find ways of obtaining exciting flavors and textures from PURE foods that were least likely to elicit a reaction. This meant cooking without dairy (milk, yogurt, butter, casein, whey), gluten, wheat, eggs, soy, peanuts, tree nuts or any type of fish or seafood. Because I wanted to keep things as natural as possible I also decided to leave out xanthum gum from the beginning.

You will find the recipes in this book use common fruits and vegetables and mostly chicken and beef in ways that are tempting to children. I use these foods to recreate a combination of old favorites in addition to coming up with fresh ideas that are designed to pass even the pickiest eater; and you can be sure that Owen has enjoyed each recipe in this book! I rely heavily on whole grain brown rice flour as my flour which is readily available by mail order as well as on tapioca starch and corn starch. If you have used whole grain brown rice flour in the past with disappointing results, do not let that sway you. I was a scientist before I was a Mom and I developed techniques to use with this flour that really make it a great base flour to use.

There are a few recipes that require noodles. I have done a thorough testing of numerous brands of rice noodles on the market and have found a version that passes my very high bar and that compliment the recipes in this book. I am proud to pass my thoughts on this in the Shortcuts and Tips section. I and everyone else I have shared them with love them.

The recipes in this book are introduced in a way that may capture the interest of a baby and toddler first (foods that are or can easily be made bite size or finger type foods) and evolve to more family style, child friendly meals toward the end. However, you know your child best so let that be your guide in picking recipes as long as your child is always supervised while eating and the foods are cut into age appropriate sizes that you are sure they can tolerate.

Lastly all the recipes in this book are designed to be quick and easy as I know what it is like to have a hungry child grabbing at your leg. This is the main reason I leave yeast out of all recipes with the exception of the Yummy Yum Little Breads Recipe. There is no yeast in the pizza dough or in the dinner rolls. Most recipes are designed for last minute preparation and can be whipped up in minutes. Along with being YUMMY and tempting to babies, toddlers and children, this was an absolute requirement. I hope they will bring smiles to your table and that you as parents become empowered by simple, pure and natural home cooking.

What this book offers:

Main Meal Focus without sacrificing dessert Yumminess

Children love dessert, however, there are at least three meals in the day that need to be filled first. This is why there is a much higher ratio of main meals to desserts in this book. Though the desserts are YUMMY and there are many recipes for the desserts we all loved growing up.

Flexibility and customizable

If your child is not allergic to all the food allergens that are entirely left out of this book you can still customize the recipes to your own children's food allergies by following some tips in the Shortcuts and Tips section.

Suitability

There is NO dairy (yogurt, butter, ice cream, casein, whey), wheat, gluten, eggs, soy, peanuts, tree nuts, seafood or xanthum gum in this book. This makes it an appropriate option for babies, toddlers and children who cannot have these foods. It is also appropriate for children with celiac disease or children who are on a casein and gluten free diet. Though please consult your child's allergist regarding the foods that are used in this book as each child's allergies are unique. Fruits, vegetables and meats can easily be substituted with those your child can have.

Nutrition

Fruits, vegetables and grains are used in ways to make them appealing to children and yummy. At the bottom of each recipe I include a simple way to highlight the nutrition in each recipe for parents.

For example, tomato * carrot * potato * corn * rice placed below a recipe means the recipe contains fruit (tomato), vegetables (carrot, potato), and grains (corn and rice). Note that this does not quantify the fruits, vegetable and grains in each recipe and does not indicate how many servings are in each recipe.

Small portions

I have opted to make the portions in this book small versus large for most recipes as they are made for young children and I have found in practice it is much easier to scale up a recipe (just double or triple everything) than it is to scale down.

Tricks and Short Cuts

This book includes a Shortcuts and Tips section in the beginning as well as Tip Boxes throughout. The latter adds layers to the book and provides you with more bang for each recipe.

Shortcuts and Tips

Precooking simple chicken and beef

Many of the recipes in the beginning and middle portion of the book require a cooked meat as a starting material. I found it much easier to precook a roast chicken (see chicken recipe on page 26) or ground beef each week that could then be stored and ready on hand for quick use in these recipes. I would refrigerate a portion for use within a couple of days and freeze the remainder. Before adding either to any of the recipes in this book I would take the *moist* portion of the chicken or beef and grind well between my fingers. This allowed these recipes to be made on hand in a snap!

Store bought vegetable and fruit purees

When a recipe calls for cooked vegetable puree such as carrot or squash I use baby food as my source as it is so easily available. Make sure you choose a brand with a single ingredient (just the vegetable) and always check the ingredient list on the back label to make sure there are no hidden other ingredients.

Check ingredient labels for everything

I am amazed at what can be hidden in the most simple of foods. I learned a lesson with tomato sauce. Make sure to check ingredient labels on *everything* to ensure that it does not contain ingredients your child may be allergic to. This should be true for all pre-bought items that you are using in recipes. I look for the products that have labels with the most basic ingredients. Do not forget to check base materials such as flour, starches, rice milk, shortening or margarine, cereals as well as ketchup, jams, herbs, vanilla extract and cocoa. Regarding the latter, you can purchase pure cocoa but watch out for powders that contain milk or milk proteins (casein, whey). It is also important to check meats, especially if they are deli meats that use a lactic acid starter culture, which can be derived from milk unless stated otherwise.

To be sure something is gluten free it should be specifically stated on the package and this includes all the base materials mentioned above and can be true for meat. If you are not sure call the company. There is one recipe in this book that calls for using *certified* gluten free oat flour (that can be made by pulverizing *certified* gluten free oats in your blender). For oats I would particularly require they are certified gluten free as crops can be contaminated with wheat from neighboring crops. You can find these online by typing "certified gluten free oats" into a search engine on the internet.

Keep it interesting

Try offering for breakfast a hardier lunch or dinner food that contains meat or for dinner try a breakfast recipe to keep things interesting.

Follow the recipes as stated

Especially in recipes that use whole grain brown rice flour you will find that they include a step that requires boiling water, rice milk or a vegetable puree that is then added to the rice flour immediately. This process is there to remove graininess from the rice flour and is an important step in the recipe. Similarly, any recipe that calls for microwaving dough as part of the preparation serves this same purpose and should be followed as directed.

There are also recipes that call for using apple cider vinegar. The vinegar is there to bring a dough or batter to an appropriate pH. Keep in mind, if this is left out it will alter the batter or dough's properties.

Shortcuts and Tips

Vegetable shortening or Margarine

In most recipes that require shortening or margarine I say that they can be used interchangeably. That is because while there is margarine available made only from vegetable oil (no other ingredient) it may be hard to find. Vegetable shortening (I use a palm shortening) is essentially the same as margarine as it is solidified oil. Just keep in mind that for these recipes, margarine will often contain salt whereas shortening will not. Depending on which one is used you may be required to alter the salt content to your liking.

White rice noodles really do noodles justice

I had the idea of replacing traditional spaghetti with white rice spaghetti immediately as I loved rice noodles in chicken soups or in Asian dishes as I child and thought they would work great with tomato sauce too. It even occurred to me that I would not feel deprived of gluten containing pasta if I could replace it with this type of noodle! I put this idea on the back burner, however, out of concern that they would have to be obtained from non-dedicated facilities out of the United States. Thankfully after several unsatisfied tries with brown rice pastas I decided to search for white rice spaghetti on the internet and found that there are sources that are made in the US or Canada in dedicated allergy free facilities! And they did not disappoint my very high bar! I like to cook them al dente and place them immediately in a bowl of cold water to stop the cooking process. This also serves to wash them well before eating. Recommendation of specific brands I have used can be found on the Yummyyumforeveryone.com website.

Homemade baking powder recipe

For all the recipes requiring baking powder in this book I recommend you make your own.

Mix ½ cup Cream of Tarter with ¼ cup baking soda and store in a sealed container.

Substitution options

If your child is not allergic to all foods left out of this book and you would like to substitute back in, keep in mind the following: applesauce or cooked carrot puree is used as an egg replacement in dessert foods so you can substitute back in where appropriate (3 Tablespoons applesauce or cooked carrot puree = 1 egg); whole grain brown rice flour is a main flour used in this book but mostly in combination with tapioca or corn starch and in some cases instant potato flakes. If your child has no problem with wheat or gluten you can try to substitute all purpose flour and replace the entire rice flour, starch and potato flake portion of the recipe. Rice milk is used in this book though you can substitute soy or dairy milk if your child is not allergic to them.

Muffin Pans

I use muffin pans in the instructions to make the Yummy Yum Little Breads, Dinner Rolls and Brownies. The only reason for this is gluten free breads and some desserts tend to sink in larger, more traditional sized pans. While there are smaller non traditional sized pans available online that may work for these recipes I have found that the most fun, convenient and easy to find tool for everyone to use is a muffin pan so I adapted the recipes to this. And you will be amazed at how much fun it is to cut open a Yummy Yum Little Bread and have a circle shaped sandwich! Though keep in mind you can always try smaller pans if you can find them and adjust times appropriately.

Nutrition Tree

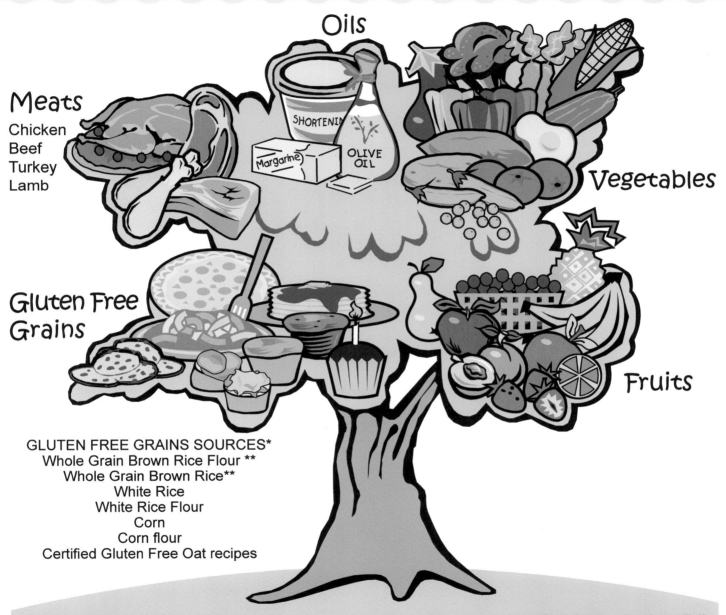

Oils

Meats
Chicken
Beef
Turkey
Lamb

Vegetables

Gluten Free Grains

Fruits

GLUTEN FREE GRAINS SOURCES*
Whole Grain Brown Rice Flour **
Whole Grain Brown Rice**
White Rice
White Rice Flour
Corn
Corn flour
Certified Gluten Free Oat recipes

*Additional Gluten Free Grain options that are not used in this book include Amaranth, Millet, Quinoa, Sorghum, Teff
** A grain is considered Whole grain when all three parts – bran, germ and endosperm – are present.

Shakes

Orange Creamsicle

4 ounces of frozen
   concentrated orange juice
1 cup rice milk
1 Tablespoon sugar
1 cup ice cubes

Mix all ingredients in a blender.
Serve immediately.

Banana Shake

1 cup rice milk (chilled)
1 ripe banana
1 Tablespoon sugar

Mix all
ingredients in a
blender. Serve
immediately.

Chocolate Carrot

¾ cup rice milk (chilled)
¼ cup cooked carrot puree
   (chilled)
½ teaspoon pure cocoa powder
1 teaspoon sugar

Place all ingredients in a cup that
has a lid. Cover and shake well.

Juicy Soda

Add a ¼ cup of your child's favorite juice (concentrated is best)
to ½ cup of seltzer water. Make sure both are chilled.

Dips

Awesome Avocado Dip

3 peeled and pitted avocados
juice of 1 lime
1 teaspoon salt
½ cup diced onion
3 Tablespoons chopped cilantro
2 diced plum tomatoes

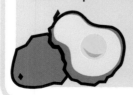

Mash the avocado.
Add lime juice, salt,
onion and cilantro.
Mix in tomatoes.

White Bean Dip

1 can (15 ounce) cannellini beans
2 Tablespoons lemon juice
⅓ cup olive oil
¼ cup fresh parsley
2 cloves of garlic
salt and pepper to taste

Add all ingredients to a food
processor. Pulse until
well mixed.

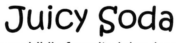

Corn Tortilla Sandwiches

This is great for older children. Coat a frying pan with a small amount of vegetable shortening or margarine and add corn tortilla. Cook open for 1 minute, add inside ingredients to one side and fold in half. Cook for 30 seconds on each side. Allow to cool. Drain on a paper towel before serving.

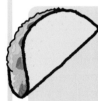

Suggested fillings:

Turkey slices and tomato
Roast chicken, bacon and tomato
Shredded steak and onion
Mini hamburgers with ketchup

Rice Cake Pizzas

When simple and quick is what you need this opens the door to so many options. Lightly coat rice cake with a small amount of pizza sauce or other appropriate sauce. Make sure it is a thin coating because too much sauce will make the rice cake soggy. Sprinkle on meat and salt or seasoning to taste. Bake at 250°F for 10 to 15 minutes on a cookie sheet.

Suggested toppings:

Tomato sauce with cooked ground beef
BBQ sauce with chicken
Mashed potato and bacon (I would still
add a thin layer of tomato sauce)

Un-Granola Mix

Lightly grind 1 rice cake plus a ½ cup of corn flakes in a blender. Place mixture in a bowl. Add ¼ cup of raisins or dried cranberries. Add 1 Tablespoon of maple syrup, ½ Tablespoon canola oil and ½ teaspoon brown sugar. Mix all ingredients well with a spoon. Evenly spread out mixture baking sheet and bake at 325°F for 10 minutes. Use two spatulas and do your best to turn mixture over. Bake an additional 5 to 10 minutes or until mixture starts to darken slightly. Remove from heat and place in a bowl. Mixture will become crispy as it cools.

Rice Cakes with Jams or Dips

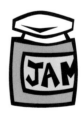

It's hard to believe I didn't consider this option until late in the game which is why I make sure to mention it here. Rice cakes are such a great way to serve jam or with dips such as the Avocado or White Bean Dip.

7

Crepe Pancakes

The secret to these pancakes is making an extremely thin crepe-like batter which makes the pancakes moist. The oil added to the batter makes them chewy and crispy at the edges.

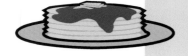

¼ cup whole grain brown rice flour
¼ cup + 1 Tablespoon corn starch or tapioca starch
½ teaspoon baking powder (recipe page 4)
2½ Tablespoons maple syrup
2½ Tablespoons canola oil
¼ cup + 2½ Tablespoons rice milk
oil or vegetable shortening to coat pan

* whole grain brown rice *

Add all dry ingredients to a bowl. Mix well.

Add remaining ingredients to the same bowl and mix again. Remember batter will be extremely thin. This consistency is necessary so do not try to make batter thicker. Lightly coat the entire bottom of a small pan with melted shortening or margarine. If there is excess, be sure to pour additional liquid off so that the pan is only lightly coated. Be sure to choose a pan size that you would like your pancake to be as the thin batter will fill the entire bottom of the pan and form a single pancake. Place pan over medium heat and pour in batter until there is just enough batter to coat the bottom. Pancake should be thin. As the pancake cooks you will see many small bubbles form on top, starting at the edges moving in. You will also notice the top of the pancake starting to look "cooked." The pancake is ready to be turned over when you see this as well as when the edges start to look crispy. Cook until golden brown.

Tip

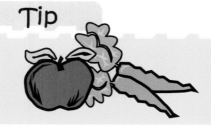

For apple or carrot pancakes, add 2½ Tablespoons applesauce or cooked carrot puree and reduce rice milk to a ¼ cup.

Rice is Nice Dishes

Perfectly simple rice dishes that have great flavor and can grow with your child.

Creamy Chicken and Broccoli Rice

½ cup cooked white rice
¼ cup cooked broccoli
2 Tablespoons cooked moist chicken
　　(grind finely between your fingers)
2 Tablespoons vegetable shortening or margarine
salt to taste

　　　　* broccoli * white rice *

Tomato-ee Beef and Rice

½ cup cooked white rice
4 Tablespoons of tomato sauce
2 Tablespoons cooked carrot puree
2 Tablespoons cooked ground beef
salt to taste
oregano to taste (optional)

　　* tomato * carrot * white rice *

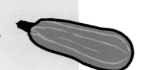

Squash and Ground Beef Rice

½ cup cooked white rice
3 Tablespoons of cooked squash puree
2 Tablespoons cooked ground beef
1 Tablespoon water
1½ teaspoon onion (optional)
salt to taste

　　　　* squash * onion * white rice *

Cook rice as usual but keep a bit moist. Add rice to a new pan. Add all remaining ingredients (this will depend on which recipe you are making above) to this pan. Mix with rice and cook over low heat for 1 to 2 minutes. Use a fork to break up any pieces of meat or vegetable. Rice dishes should have a smooth creamy consistency.

Squash Beef Cakes

Owen would clap his hands when he saw this was for lunch or dinner. Serve with extra maple syrup on the side for dipping. You may sprinkle with additional salt after cooking. Makes 6 to 8 quarter size cakes.

3 Tablespoons whole grain brown rice flour
½ Tablespoon corn flour
1½ Tablespoons corn starch or tapioca starch
4 Tablespoons cooked ground beef
3 Tablespoons cooked squash puree
2 Tablespoons maple syrup
¼ teaspoon salt
canola oil for frying

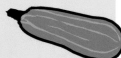

* squash * corn * whole grain brown rice *

Chicken Carrot Cakes

This recipe is the same idea as the Squash Beef Cakes but with a great chicken and carrot combination. Alternatively cooked ground beef can be used to replace the chicken in this recipe. Serve with ketchup for dipping. You may sprinkle with additional salt after cooking. Makes 6 to 8 quarter size cakes.

3 Tablespoons whole grain brown rice flour
½ Tablespoon corn flour
1½ Tablespoons corn starch or tapioca starch
4 Tablespoons cooked moist chicken
   (grind finely between your fingers)
5 Tablespoons cooked carrot puree
Up to 5 Tablespoons water
¼ teaspoon onion powder
¼ teaspoon salt
canola oil for frying

* carrot * corn * whole grain brown rice *

Add all ingredients *except* the appropriate vegetable puree (this will depend on which of the above recipes you are making) or water (only if you are making the chicken carrot cake recipe) to a bowl. Then bring the appropriate puree to quick boil in a pan over medium heat. Immediately remove heated puree and add to a bowl containing all other ingredients. Mix quickly. This process will remove any graininess in the rice flour. Batter should be slightly wet but not runny. In the case of the chicken carrot cakes you will need to add up to 5 Tablespoons of water to achieve the correct consistency. If you are unsure, add 2½ Tablespoons and try cooking a small batch to test. The batter should be moist but when cooked should not fall apart. The middle should cook entirely and the outside should brown nicely and be slightly crisp. Add oil to bottom of pan so that it is approximately a ¼ inch deep and place pan over medium heat. Use a Tablespoon to scoop out batter and dollop into pan one cake at a time. Cook over medium heat and turn regularly until all sides are medium brown. Place on a paper towel to drain.

Chicken and Broccoli French Fries

This is toddler proof in every way and is a great way to hide vegetables and meat. This can be made with any store bought French fries or sweet potato fries as well as Homemade Mashed Potato Fries on page 24. Serve with ketchup on the side.

Frozen French fries
½ cup whole grain brown rice flour
¼ teaspoon garlic powder
¼ teaspoon onion powder
¼ teaspoon salt
Up to a ¾ cup of water (probably will use close
    to ½ cup or slightly over)
4 Tablespoons moist cooked chicken
    (grind finely between your fingers)
3 Tablespoons well cooked broccoli florets
canola oil for frying

* broccoli * onion * potato or sweet potato *
whole grain brown rice *

Add flour, garlic powder, onion powder and salt to a large bowl. Mix well. Add chicken and broccoli and mix again. Gradually stir in enough water so that the mixture is a wet paste. It should be wet but thick enough to grab onto and thickly coat the French fries during the coating process. Add oil to the bottom of pan so that it is approximately a ¼ inch deep and place over medium to high heat. Dip each French fry individually into bowl, cover thickly with batter and immediately place in pan. French fries should be placed evenly apart so they do not stick together. Fry and turn over repeatedly until golden brown on all sides. Remove immediately and drain on paper towels.

Tip

If you would like to use homemade French fries instead of store bought make sure they are sliced very thin to allow thorough cooking inside. Store bought French fries have the advantage of being precooked and this ensures they will be cooked entirely in this recipe.

Tomato Soup

This is so simple and goes great with chicken nuggets.
It also served as a base sauce for the No Noodle Lasagna recipe found at the end of this section (page 36).

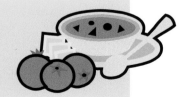

1 cup tomato juice
½ cup cooked carrot puree
salt to taste
pepper to taste

* tomato * carrot *

Add tomato juice and carrot puree to a pan and bring up to medium heat. Allow to simmer approximately 5 minutes until thickened. Remove from heat. Add salt and pepper to taste.

Yummy Yum Little Breads

Little breads are made in muffin pans and are soft, chewy with a slight oat taste. Slice them in half and they are perfect for sandwiches. Use an oven thermometer to ensure appropriate oven temperature, critical for cooking breads, especially small breads. Makes 12 little breads.

Proofing Yeast

3 teaspoons gluten free Active Dry Yeast (not heaping)
¾ cup rice milk
3 Tablespoons sugar

Add ¾ cup of rice milk to a small bowl. Microwave until liquid is just warm to touch but not hot. Mix in sugar. Stir to dissolve. Add yeast to this same bowl. Let yeast sit on top of rice milk for 30 seconds and then start to mix yeast. If clumps form, remove them and continue to mix remaining yeast (I found there will still be sufficient yeast left over). Cover with a kitchen towel and set aside in a warm place (I put on top of the clothes dryer while it is running) for 15 to 30 minutes or until yeast creates a foamy layer on top of the liquid (this shows it is active, if it does not become foamy you must restart with new yeast).

Bread Ingredients

1½ cup whole grain brown rice flour
¾ cup *certified* gluten free oats (pulverize first in blender to form a flour)
1 cup plus 2½ Tablespoons tapioca starch
¼ cup plus 2½ Tablespoons corn starch
3 teaspoons unflavored gelatin (not heaping)
¾ teaspoon salt
6 Tablespoons applesauce
6 Tablespoons melted vegetable shortening (measure after melting)

* apple * whole grain brown rice * oat *

Make sure all bread ingredients are at room temperature prior to starting. Bring oven to 200°F (use an oven thermometer to ensure accurate temperate which is critical for bread). Turn oven off when the dough is mixed as it will be used to allow bread dough to rise. Add all the dry bread ingredients to a large bowl. Mix well. Add applesauce and melted shortening. Mix well again. Add entire yeast liquid (⅓ of volume at a time), including the foamy portion and mix with your hands for 5 minutes until yeast is fully mixed in. Dough will be wet but will thicken slightly with mixing. Grease all the wells in a muffin pan. Fill wells half way up with dough. Cover with saran wrap. Place pan in oven on middle rack and allow it to rise at 200°F (remember oven should be turned off just before placing in). When dough has risen to the top of the wells, remove from oven and set aside. Note, the rising process could take up to 45 minutes to an hour. Heat oven to 350°F. Bake bread UNCOVERED for 9 minutes on middle rack, and then COVERED with aluminum foil for an additional 5 to 7 minutes or until lightly browned. Allow to cool 5 minutes and then remove from pan. *While bread is still warm* place immediately in a ziplock bag. If you would like to keep beyond 4 hours, slice breads and *while bread is still warm* freeze immediately in a ziplock bag. To thaw, just remove bag from freezer and allow to thaw at room temperature in a sealed ziplock bag. They will be ready for lunch if removed in the morning!

Sweet French Toast

This is just like the French Toast you grew up on. For an extra treat serve with powdered sugar or your child's favorite fruit. Makes up to 6 medium size pieces of French Toast.

Yummy Yum Little Breads (recipe page 12)
   or your favorite bread
¼ cup tapioca starch
3 Tablespoons applesauce
3 Tablespoons rice milk
2 Tablespoons maple syrup
½ teaspoon vanilla extract (optional)
margarine or vegetable shortening for frying

 * apple * whole grain brown rice * oat *

Add all ingredients to a bowl. Mix well. Lightly coat a frying pan with melted margarine or shortening. Quickly dip each side of bread into the bowl allowing both sides to be coated. However, bread should not be submerged completely into liquid as bread will become soggy. Allow excess liquid to drip off bread or wipe excess off with your fingers before placing in frying pan over medium heat. Cook as you would any French toast. Turn regularly until nicely browned on both sides. Note that it may take longer to brown than traditional French Toast but it will brown nicely if you cook it long enough. I like to press down on the bread with the spatula periodically to ensure good contact with the surface of the pan.

Tip

French Toast is perfect for making Monte Cristo or Reuben style sandwiches.

Beef Stroganoff Noodles

*Ketchup gives a hint of extra flavor to this dish. Boiling down rice milk adds a nice creaminess.
This is a great dish to add vegetables your child likes to eat such as corn, peas or broccoli.*

1 cup al dente cooked white rice spaghetti
  (see Shortcuts and Tips Section page 4)
4 Tablespoons uncooked ground beef
½ cup of water
½ cup rice milk
½ teaspoon salt
1 teaspoon ketchup

* tomato * optional vegetables * white rice *

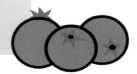

Add water and uncooked meat to a pan. Cook meat over medium heat. When meat is almost cooked and the majority of liquid has boiled away, add rice milk, salt and al dente cooked noodles. Stir continuously and allow the majority of rice milk to boil away (1 to 2 minutes). When this occurs remove pan from heat and add ketchup.

Creamy Tomato Sauce Noodles

As with the stroganoff dish above boiling down rice milk makes the tomato sauce rich and creamy.

1 cup al dente cooked white rice spaghetti
  (see Shortcuts and Tips Section page 4)
4 Tablespoons uncooked ground beef
½ cup water
½ teaspoon salt
⅓ cup tomato sauce
½ cup rice milk

* tomato * optional vegetables *
       white rice *

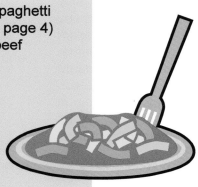

Add water and uncooked meat to a pan. Cook meat over medium heat. When meat is almost cooked, add rice milk, salt, tomato sauce and al dente cooked noodles. Stir continuously and allow the majority of rice milk to boil away (1 to 2 minutes). Once this occurs you may remove from heat.

Pop Pop Chicken Bites

This is such a fun way to serve chicken to children and it's loaded with whole grain brown rice flour that they'll never know. The chicken comes out moist on the inside and crispy on the outside. Serve with ketchup or your favorite sauce on the side.

⅔ cup uncooked chicken cutlet that has been
   chopped in blender
⅓ cup rice milk
¼ cup plus 2 Tablespoons whole grain brown rice flour
½ teaspoon of salt
additional salt to taste (after frying)
canola oil for frying

* whole grain brown rice *

Place chicken in a blender and allow blender to chop or grind into small pieces. Note, some chicken will stick together and pieces will be variable in size. This is fine as larger pieces will be broken into smaller pieces while cooking. Measure out ⅔ cup of chopped chicken and place in a bowl. Pour in rice milk. Allow rice milk to coat chicken and then pour off excess rice milk. Mix flour and salt together in a separate bowl. Now add the flour and salt mixture to the bowl containing the chicken. Mix well to coat the chicken.

Add oil to bottom of frying pan so that it is approximately ¼ inch deep and bring over medium heat. Add chicken to pan. As chicken is cooking break up any large pieces that may stick together so chicken can cook thoroughly. Pieces should be approximately popcorn size, some slightly bigger or smaller. Turn chicken frequently and allow chicken to cook until it is medium brown on the outside, starts to get crispy in places and is cooked thoroughly on the inside. Place chicken on a paper towel and allow to drain.

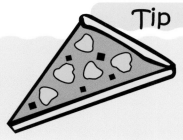

Tip

This is a great pizza topping (pages 18 and 28) with tomato sauce and also works well as a chicken source in the Breaded Italian Chicken Bites recipe (pages 31).

BBQ Chicken

This is such a simple BBQ sauce. For the flavors to come out fully it requires baking with chicken that contains both skin and bone. The juices of the chicken then come together for a complete BBQ sauce.

4 uncooked chicken parts containing bone and skin
2 Tablespoons apricot or peach jam
2 Tablespoons ketchup
2 Tablespoons tomato paste
2 Tablespoons canola oil
1 teaspoon onion powder
2 teaspoons brown sugar
⅔ teaspoon salt

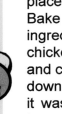

* apricot or peach * tomato * white rice (optional) *

Preheat oven to 350°F. In an oven safe dish place chicken side by side so that it fits snugly. Bake for 25 minutes uncovered. Mix all remaining ingredients in a bowl to form sauce. Remove chicken from oven and pour sauce over chicken and coat chicken on all sides. Turn chicken upside down so that it is now on the opposite side of what it was when cooking previously and place back in oven (crispy side down). Bake uncovered for an additional 20 to 25 minutes or until chicken is cooked thoroughly on the inside.

Tip

For older children this is great to serve with French fries. For younger children try "pulling" the inside meat of the chicken and add to white rice along with some of the leftover BBQ sauce. Heat briefly in a pan to combine flavors.

Oven Baked Drumsticks

This tastes just like the baked chicken I grew up on. Try this recipe with small chicken wing size drumsticks for fun.

4 uncooked chicken legs with skin
1 cup rice milk
1 cup whole grain brown rice flour
⅓ cup vegetable shortening or margarine
salt to taste

* whole grain brown rice *

Preheat oven to 375°F. Place shortening or margarine in an oven safe dish. Place in the oven and allow to melt. Make sure the dish you choose will fit the size of your chicken snugly as you want to make sure there is sufficient vegetable shortening or margarine remaining at the bottom of the dish through the cooking process. Meanwhile dip chicken in rice milk and then in flour until fully coated. Place chicken on top of melted shortening or margarine in dish. Cook for 20 minutes and turn chicken over. Cook an additional 45 to 50 minutes or until juices run clear and chicken is nicely browned. Allow chicken to drain on paper towels.

Tip

For younger children this can be cut up into very small pieces or for older children is great just served with rice and salad on the side.

16

Toddler Friendly Stuffing

This hamburger stuffing was a sure bet during the picky eater stage. Yummy Yum Little Breads work great with this recipe. The stuffing is moist enough to be made into little ball shapes for small hands just before serving.

1¼ cup Yummy Yum Little Breads pulled into cubes (page 12) or your favorite bread
3 Tablespoons cooked ground beef
¾ teaspoon ketchup
¼ teaspoon parsley (optional)
1 Tablespoon margarine or vegetable shortening
salt to taste

apple (if you are using Yummy Yum Little Breads) *
tomato * whole grain brown rice *

Heat margarine or shortening in a pan over medium heat. Toss in bread cubes and turn bread regularly until lightly browned on all sides, approximately 2 to 4 minutes. Add ketchup and stir an additional 1 to 2 minutes. Remove from heat. Add cooked beef and parsley. Add salt to taste. Serve warm. If stuffing dries out you can rehydrate with a small amount of water.

Turkey Sausage Patties

I could never trust store bought sausage with all the different ingredients so I set out to make my own homemade sausage that could be whipped up in minutes. Shape into small links or patties. Makes 8 to 10.

1 cup uncooked ground white turkey meat
¾ Tablespoon oregano
¾ teaspoon thyme
½ teaspoon ginger
½ teaspoon paprika
½ teaspoon salt
¼ teaspoon ground pepper
canola oil for coating pan

Mix all ingredients in a bowl. Form into patties or links. Lightly coat a pan with oil over medium heat. Add sausage and allow to cook over medium to high heat. Turn frequently until nicely browned and sausages are no longer pink in the center. This will take between 10 and 15 minutes.

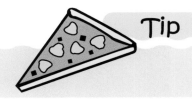

Tip

This sausage is perfect crumbled up and served as a pizza topping!

17

Mashed Potato Pizza

To help with the picky eater stage the toppings are added to the inside of the mashed potato pizza. An enticing crispy layer is formed on the top of the pizza by drizzling a light coating of melted vegetable shortening or margarine during the baking process. Try these suggested pizzas or come up with your own creations – there are so many options.

1 cup instant mashed potato flakes
½ cup rice milk (boiled)
¼ teaspoon salt (if you use salted margarine to coat the top of the pizza you may not need to add salt)
Up to 3 Tablespoons vegetable shortening or margarine (to coat top of pizza)

Beef and Tomato

2½ Tablespoons tomato sauce
2½ Tablespoons cooked carrot puree
⅓ cup cooked beef
oregano to taste (optional)

Turkey Sausage and Tomato

¼ cup tomato sauce
⅓ cup cooked turkey sausage (crumble sausage with fingers) (recipe page 17)

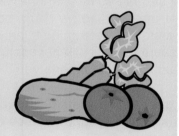

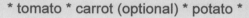
* tomato * carrot (optional) * potato *

Preheat oven to 375°F. Mix potato flakes and salt. Bring rice milk to a quick boil and immediately remove from heat and add to bowl containing potato flakes and salt. Depending on which pizza you are making, add appropriate meat and sauce. Mix well. Spread potato dough *thinly* into an aluminum pan with sides. I like to use a small spring form pan (do not use a pizza stone as dough will stick). Pour melted shortening or margarine over pizza. Pour off any remaining shortening or margarine as excess liquid should not pool on pizza and should only coat the top to make it crispy. Bake for 20 to 30 minutes or until top becomes nicely browned and crispy.

Tip

Try adding pulled BBQ chicken and sauce from page 16 or pulled chicken from the baked chicken drumsticks on page 18 (be sure to include some of the breading from the chicken pieces because it will add such flavor; crumple it into small pieces prior to adding). Cooked carrot puree can be used as a sauce as it pairs well with the baked chicken drumsticks in this pizza recipe.

Vegetable French Toast

Vegetable purees are used to make a batter to coat bread and then the bread is cooked just like the traditional sweet form of French toast. This actually works well with store bought gluten free rice bread as it enhances chewiness and gives a savory flavor. This is a great snack and fun for cutting into shapes.

Broccoli and Tomato

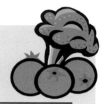

2 Tablespoons cooked broccoli puree
1 Tablespoon tomato sauce

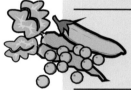

Pea and Carrot

2 Tablespoons cooked pea puree
1 Tablespoon cooked carrot puree

Tomato and Basil

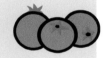

2 Tablespoons tomato sauce
⅓ teaspoon chopped fresh basil

* optional vegetables * whole grain brown rice *

If using frozen bread briefly warm in oven or microwave first. Mix appropriate purees in a bowl. Using your fingers, coat bread on both sides as if painting the bread until it is fully coated on both sides. Do not overly coat and do not dip bread. Add only enough of the mixture to "color" the bread or bread will become soggy. Note you will likely have some of the mixture leftover. Coat frying pan with a small amount of shortening or margarine by bringing up to medium heat. Pour off any excess oil and leave only enough to form a light coat. Add coated bread to pan. Turn frequently until browned on both sides. Allow to sit on paper towel to remove excess oil.

Tip

For an alternative pizza crust or as a bread base for hamburgers, meatloaf sandwiches, cold cuts, or the bread base of sloppy joes, try frying bread in just shortening or margarine alone. This will make the bread crispy and it will add flavor and texture to the bread.

Sweet Potato Chip Tacos

The flavors of sweet potato and seasoned taco meat work really well together. This is a recipe which requires a special tool to slice potatoes called a mandolin which is necessary to slice potatoes thin enough to get them crispy.

Sweet Potato Chips

sweet potatoes cut with a mandolin
   (sliced on the thinnest setting)
canola oil for frying

Taco Meat

½ cup cooked ground beef
3 Tablespoons cooked carrot puree
3 Tablespoons tomato sauce
¼ teaspoon onion powder
¼ teaspoon garlic powder
¼ teaspoon paprika (optional)
1/8 teaspoon chili powder (optional)

* tomato * sweet potato * carrot *

To obtain good crispiness for making these chips requires two steps. First the thinly sliced potatoes are lightly fried. They are then baked at a low temperature on a baking sheet.

Add enough oil to the bottom of frying pan so that it is approximately ¼ inch deep. Bring up to high heat for 1 minute. Add sweet potato slices and spread them out around the pan and continue to cook over high heat for 1 to 2 minutes. Make sure they are submerged in oil. You will begin to see the actual potatoes bubbling a bit. Once this occurs, remove the slices from the oil and place on a paper towel. Note it is important to remove them before they start to burn as they have a high sugar content and can burn easily. Pat dry.

Preheat oven to 250°F. Place sliced potatoes evenly apart on a cookie sheet. Place in oven and bake for 10 minutes. Turn slices over and bake an additional 10 minutes or until crispy. Remove from oven and place briefly on a paper towel and then move to a plate.

Mix all ingredients in a pan and cook over low to medium heat for 1 to 2 minutes. Allow to thicken and then remove from heat. Place Taco Meat in the center of a plate and place the sweet potato chips around the edges of the plate for dipping.

20

Yummy Yum Quick Dinner Rolls

The simplest bread possible, these are yummy as snacks and can be served with margarine and are also great with jam. Makes 5 dinner rolls.

½ cup whole grain brown rice flour
¼ cup instant mashed potato flakes
¼ cup tapioca starch
2½ Tablespoons corn starch
1 teaspoon baking powder (see page 4)
1 teaspoon sugar
2 Tablespoons olive oil
1 Tablespoon applesauce
½ cup water

* potato * whole grain brown rice *

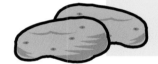

Preheat oven to 375°F. Start bringing water to a quick boil. This is a necessary step to remove graininess from flour.

Add all dry ingredients to a bowl and mix well. Add oil and applesauce. Once water is boiled add it immediately to bowl containing all the ingredients. Mix well but quickly to form dough. Dough will be light and airy. Lightly grease wells of a cupcake pan and loosely place dough into each well. Fill each well to just a bit more than half the well depth. Do not pat dough down to fit extra dough in well, it is important that it remains "light" in the well.

Bake for 20 to 25 minutes or until top becomes lightly browned. Allow to cool briefly and slice open. If you are not going to serve immediately, place rolls in ziplock bags (*while still warm*) for a couple of hours to prevent drying out. You may also freeze rolls (*while still warm*) in ziplock bags for later use. To thaw, allow rolls to sit at room temperature while they remain in a ziplock bag.

Chicken or Turkey Nuggets

The secret here is the uncooked nuggets are dipped in corn starch bath as an egg replacer and then they are dipped in the breading. The nuggets are then fried in a small amount of oil just to "set" the breading and then they are baked.

Bowl 1 – Corn starch bath

1 Tablespoon corn starch
¼ cup water

Bowl 2 - Breading Coating

2 Tablespoons whole grain brown
2 Tablespoons white rice flour
1 Tablespoons Tapioca starch
½ teaspoon sugar
1/3 teaspoon salt

Additional

1 skinless chicken or turkey breast
   (uncooked and cut into nugget
   size pieces)
bowl of water to place uncooked
   nuggets
canola oil for frying
salt to taste

* whole grain brown rice *

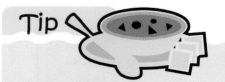

Tip

These nuggets are great for chicken cutlet sandwiches or paired with tomato soup.

In Bowl 1 mix the corn starch and water to create the <u>Corn starch bath</u> (note you may have to stir regularly to keep the corn starch from falling to the bottom). In BOWL 2 mix all the ingredients under <u>Breading Coating</u> ingredient list. Add all uncooked nuggets to the separate bowl of water to get them initially moist. Remove one nugget from the water (work with one piece at a time) and quickly dip nugget into BOWL 1 to coat in the corn starch bath, then very quickly dip the same piece into the place into BOWL 2 for the breading coating. Make sure the chicken is coated thoroughly in this final step though I do *not* recommend letting the nuggets "sit" in this final coating as it could dry out the nuggets by removing too much water. I prefer to remove the nuggets immediately after the last dipping step and place them on a plate until they are ready to be placed in oil. Repeat these dipping steps with the remaining pieces. They should all follow this dipping sequence: water-Corn starch bath-Final Breading Coating.

Add enough oil to a frying pan so that it is approximately ¼ inch deep. Place pan over medium to high heat. Add coated nuggets to the pan and cook briefly on all sides until the breading is "set." This should only take a total of 2 to 4 minutes. Note that excess breading may come off but there should be sufficient breading that remains. Drain well on a paper towel.

Preheat oven to 350°F. Place nuggets on a cookie sheet and cook for 20 minutes or until the inside the nuggets are thoroughly cooked. You may sprinkle with additional salt prior to baking or following baking.

Do's Make sure the nuggets are drained well on a paper towel (both sides of the nuggets) after frying and prior to baking.

Do Not's Do not preheat the cookie sheet in the oven. Rather place nuggets on cookie sheet after draining on the paper towel and place in the oven at the time of baking the nuggets.
Do not turn nuggets during the baking process. Allow them to bake the entire way the same way you placed them on the cookie sheet.

Quick Gnocchi with Creamy Tomato Carrot Sauce

This a terrific Italian potato pasta and is a great place to put in your child's favorite vegetables. It also makes a great baked pasta dish if you like. Don't let making gnocchi homemade scare you, it is so simple and is done in 15 minutes. Makes approximately 3 cups of gnocchi.

Gnocchi
2 cups instant mashed potato flakes
2 cups boiling water
2 Tablespoons margarine, melted
2 teaspoons salt
flour mix* (premix 2 cups whole grain
   brown rice flour + 1½ cups tapioca starch
   + ½ cup corn starch)

Sauce
1 cup tomato sauce
½ cup cooked carrot puree
⅓ cup uncooked ground beef
½ teaspoon garlic salt
1 cup water
optional cooked vegetables
   (broccoli, peas, green beans, spinach)

* tomato * carrot * potato * whole grain brown rice *

Place potato flakes in a medium size bowl. Pour in boiling water; stir until blended. Stir in margarine and salt. Let cool. Blend in enough flour mixture to make a fairly stiff dough, approximately 3 cups. Turn dough out on a well floured board. Knead lightly. Pull off some dough and form into a thin roll, the thickness of a thin breadstick. With a knife dipped in flour, cut into bite-size pieces, keep in mind gnocchi will expand while boiling.

Bring a large volume of water to boiling in a pot. Place a handful gnocchi in boiling water. As the gnocchi rise to the top of the pot, remove them with a slotted spoon and place into a bowl of cold water to cool them immediately (this is also important so they do not stick together). Repeat until all are cooked. Drain gnocchi.

To prepare sauce add water and ground beef to a pan and cook over medium heat. You may add additional water if necessary until meat is thoroughly cooked. Once meat is cooked, allow remaining water to boil away. Add remaining sauce ingredients and cook for an additional three to five minutes allowing sauce to thicken slightly. Add appropriate amount of sauce to gnocchi and mix well. *There will be extra flour mix remaining.

Tips

#1 – You can try to substitute in some cooked sweet potato for a portion of the instant mashed potato flakes to give it a slightly sweet flavor. You may need to add additional flour mixture to achieve the correct consistency.

#2 – Try adding Italian seasonings to dough for extra flavor.

Homemade Mashed Potato French Fries

At some point we realized that if we could hide meat in a French fry, Owen would eat it. This was especially true during a picky eater phase. I tucked small bits of turkey or ham inside French fries prior to the baking step. Makes 16 fries.

1 cup instant mashed potato flakes
6 teaspoons oil
2 Tablespoons whole grain brown rice flour
¼ teaspoon salt
½ cup water (boiled)
canola oil for frying

Optional

Add cold cuts thinly sliced and cut into very small pieces (buy prepackaged but still be sure to check label for hidden ingredients)

* potato * whole grain brown rice *

Preheat oven to 325°F. Mix all dry ingredients except meat. Add boiled water. Form into ½ inch size potato balls and if you are inserting meat do it at this stage (make sure meat is in the center and that you reseal the French fry). Place in a glass dish (they may burn on aluminum pans) and bake for 7 to 10 minutes until slightly brown. You can freeze at this stage if you are making large batches or proceed to next step.

Add oil to the bottom of a frying pan so that it is approximately a ¼ inch deep and place on medium heat. Add French fries and turn regularly until golden brown. Remove and immediately drain on a paper towel. Serve with ketchup.

Tip

You can use these French Fries in combination with the recipe for Chicken and Broccoli French fry recipe on page 11. Just dip them in the batter after the baking step and prior to the frying step.

24

Your Favorite Meatloaf

This is great as a main meal or as a base for meatloaf sandwiches.
You can also try serving with Smashed Potatoes and Gravy (page 35).

4 cups uncooked ground beef
½ cup plus 4 Tablespoons corn flour
1 teaspoon onion powder or flakes
1 ⅓ teaspoons garlic powder
1 teaspoon salt
4 Tablespoons cooked carrot puree
½ cup ketchup

* carrot * tomato * onion
* potato (optional) *
corn * whole grain brown rice *

Preheat oven to 375°F. Add all ingredients to a bowl and mix well. Fill an appropriate size meatloaf pan and bake on middle rack uncovered for 50 to 60 minutes or until nicely browned and cooked through the center. You may want to pour off any liquid that pools in the bottom of the pan when the meatloaf has approximately 10 to 15 minutes left to cook.

Tip

If you cannot use corn flour, you can try replacing corn flour with instant mashed potato flakes.

Mini Meatballs

Made small, these are great to serve with white rice spaghetti and tomato sauce.

2 cups uncooked ground beef
½ cup instant mashed potato flakes
3 Tablespoons whole grain brown rice flour
1 Tablespoon apple cider vinegar
1½ Tablepoons parsley
¼ teaspoon garlic powder
¾ teaspoon salt
¼ cup cooked carrot puree

* carrot * potato (optional) *
whole grain brown rice *

Preheat oven to 375°F. Mix all ingredients in a bowl. Form into mini meatballs. Place on a baking sheet and cook for 5 to 8 minutes or until browned on the outside and thoroughly cooked on the inside.

Crispy Chicken and Potatoes

I really wanted to make sure that I included a great basic chicken and potato dish which is versatile for a family meal and also a great way to prepare juicy cooked chicken as a base for other dishes.

2 lbs uncooked chicken cut up into parts
   (legs, thighs, breast)
8 to 10 small red potatoes (cut into wedges)
½ cup extra virgin olive oil
1 Tablespoon chopped rosemary
1½ teaspoons chopped oregano
½ teaspoon garlic powder
salt to taste

* potato *

Preheat oven to 375°F. Place chicken and potatoes in a large casserole dish. Pour olive oil over chicken and potatoes, stir to coat. Spread chicken and potatoes evenly throughout dish. Sprinkle with salt, rosemary, oregano and garlic salt. Bake for 45 minutes. Pour off juice that may have collected at the bottom of the dish (see TIP - you can save this to make gravy for this dish). Place back in the oven for an additional 15 minutes or until chicken is fully cooked.

Tip

Try serving with gravy recipe on page 35.
You can add some liquid collected in this recipe to replace some of the chicken broth used in the gravy recipe.

Sweet and Sour Chicken Spaghetti

This is a great change when you want something different from the traditional spaghetti and tomato sauce.

1½ cup white rice spaghetti cooked al dente
(see Shortcuts and Tips Section page 4)
¼ cup apricot or peach preserves
2 teaspoons tomato paste
2½ teaspoons apple cider vinegar
2 teaspoons corn starch
2 teaspoons cooked carrot puree
1/8 teaspoon crushed red pepper flakes (optional)
½ teaspoon garlic salt
⅔ cup cooked chicken breast (boiled or roasted – grind
finely between your fingers)
salt to taste

* peach or apricot * tomato * carrot * white rice *

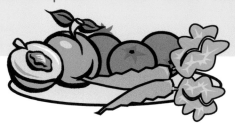

Prepare spaghetti and cook until al dente. While spaghetti is cooking mix all ingredients except chicken and salt and cook over low to medium heat for 2 to 4 minutes. Remove from heat. Add chicken to pan containing sauce and mix well. Add cooked spaghetti to pan and mix again. Add salt to taste.

27

Yummy Yum Thin Pizza Crust

The trick to this crispy thin yet chewy pizza crust is a microwave step I developed that removes graininess from the dough that is notorious with rice flours. Parchment paper is also critical to obtaining a crisp bottom. Once the dough is prepared by this method it is baked as usual. A must try to taste how good this is for yourself. Makes one oblong 8 to 10 inch length pizza, 1/8 inch in depth.

¼ cup whole grain brown rice flour
¼ cup tapioca starch
2 Tablespoons corn starch
1 Tablespoon instant mashed potato flakes
1 teaspoon baking powder (recipe page 4)
1 teaspoon apple cider vinegar
1 teaspoon Italian herbs (optional)
¼ teaspoon salt
2½ Tablespoons of canola oil
¼ cup plus 1 Tablespoon rice milk

* potato * whole grain brown rice *

Pizza Topping Ideas

Pop Pop Chicken with Tomato Sauce (page 15)

Mashed potato and Bacon

Meatloaf with Tomato Sauce (page 25)

Turkey Sausage (page 17)

Grilled Chicken with Bacon and Tomato Sauce

Ground Beef with Diced Tomatoes

Preheat oven to 450°F. Add all dry ingredients to a microwave safe *bowl* and mix well. Add remaining ingredients and mix again. Dough will be wet and runny, almost like a batter. Let sit for 5 to 10 minutes. Mix again and collect the dough together in the bottom of the bowl. Microwave on high for 30 seconds and check dough. You are looking for the dough to appear "set" on the *bottom portion* (it will not stick to your fingers when touched) though still somewhat wet to touch on the *top portion*. If dough has not achieved this then microwave at 10 to 20 second intervals until ready. Once dough is ready, remove and mix well with a spoon. You will note that upon mixing there will be additional liquid areas hidden inside the dough as there was with the top. It is important that this occurs. Mixing all areas of the dough (the "set" plus the wet portions) is important to achieve the correct consistency of the dough to proceed. At this point the dough should feel close in consistency to a gluten containing dough.

Place dough in between 2 large pieces of parchment paper. Use a large drinking glass to roll dough so that it achieves 1/8 inch thickness and is oblong in shape. It may be slightly thicker but should still remain a thin pizza.

Tip

Remove <u>top</u> parchment paper layer and form a slightly thicker crust around edges. Place pizza with parchment paper directly on rack in oven and cook for 7 minutes. Add a thin layer of sauce and toppings and bake an additional 12 to 15 minutes or until crust has begun to brown nicely.

For a more flavorful pizza dough remove 2½ Tablespoons of the rice milk portion and replace with same volume of tomato sauce. Or for a dough with a little more of a Mediterranean taste remove 2½ Tablespoons of the rice milk portion and replace with 2½ Tablespoons of water from canned olives. The water from the surrounding olives gives the dough extra flare and a nice color.

28

Corn Tortilla Gyros

A perfect dish to serve with French fries on the side. This is also a great recipe for grilling.

Gyro

1 cup uncooked ground beef
1 cup uncooked ground lamb
⅓ teaspoon salt
1 teaspoon parsley
1 teaspoon oregeno
1 Tablespoon whole grain brown flour
corn tortillas
canola oil for frying

Optional Topping

⅔ cup chopped cucumber (squeeze in a
    paper towel to remove excess water)
1½ Tablespoons vegetable shortening
¼ teaspoon salt
1 teaspoon lemon juice
pepper to taste

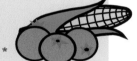

* tomato * cucumber * corn * while grain brown rice flour *

Add all ingredients for the Topping portion of the recipe in a bowl and mix well. Cover and place in refrigerator for at least a half hour to cool.

Mix all the gyro ingredients in a bowl. Shape into small patties between 1/8 and a ¼ inch thick. I like to place the patties between two pieces of parchment paper and roll over them with a glass to make them thin. Add 1 Tablespoon of canola oil to a pan, allow to coat and bring up to medium heat. Add gyros to pan and allow to cook for 2 to 3 minutes on each side or until nicely browned. You may need to add additional time to ensure the center part is cooked thoroughly. Remove from heat.

To prepare corn tortilla, I think it is better to slightly fry them in a light amount of oil on both sides and then drain on a paper towel.

You can add gyros to the tortillas while the tortillas are frying. Once they are assembled and removed from heat add a small amount of topping and serve immediately.

Tip

Freshly diced tomatoes makes an additional great topping.

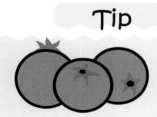

Chicken and Peppers with Vinegar

This chicken dish has so much flavor and is a great chicken parmesan substitute, just top it with tomato sauce. For older children serve with noodles or rice. For younger children cut up into very small pieces and mix with rice. If your child does not like to eat peppers, still use them in the recipe as they add great flavor and then remove for serving.

4 skinless, boneless chicken breast halves
1 cup rice milk
1 cup whole grain brown rice flour
½ cup chopped green or red or yellow peppers
¼ to ½ cup apple cider vinegar; divided
salt and pepper to taste
2 Tablespoons canola oil

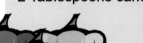

* tomato (optional) * peppers *
whole grain brown rice *

Deseed and slice peppers. If you would like to finely chop in the blender, freeze the night before and they will chop much easier. Dip chicken in rice milk and coat with brown rice flour. Add oil to pan and cook peppers over medium heat until just soft. Remove and put aside. Add 2 Tablespoons of cider vinegar to pan and add chicken. Cook for 1 to 2 minutes on each side and then add an additional ¼ cup cider vinegar to pan. Continue allowing chicken to cook, turning chicken as needed. Add additional apple cider vinegar if chicken requires more liquid to cook thoroughly. Once chicken is cooked, add back peppers and allow to cook an additional minute. Remove from heat.

Tip

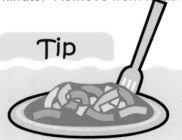

Cut the chicken into strips and serve with tomato sauce over white spaghetti noodles.

Italian Breaded Chicken Bites

*These small bites are as worthy as any appetizer served in a restaurant.
They are worth the little extra effort and they are one of my favorites.*

½ cup cooked breaded chicken from
　　Chicken and Peppers with Vinegar recipe (page 30)
　　or Pop Pop Chicken (page 15)
　　or Chicken Nuggets (page 22)
　　(chop chicken into very small pieces in blender)
¾ cup cooked white rice
3 Tablespoons whole grain brown rice flour
½ Tablespoon corn meal
¼ cup tomato sauce
¼ teaspoon salt
canola oil for frying

* tomato * peppers (optional) * whole grain brown rice *
white rice * corn *

Mix all ingredients and form into small balls. Cover the bottom of a frying pan with oil about a ¼ inch deep. Bring up to medium heat and add balls, turning frequently allowing them to brown evenly on all sides. They are cooked when they are medium brown on all sides. Allow to drain on paper towels.

31

Chicken Soup (but Not Soupy) Noodles

This is such a hearty dish that has children written all over it.

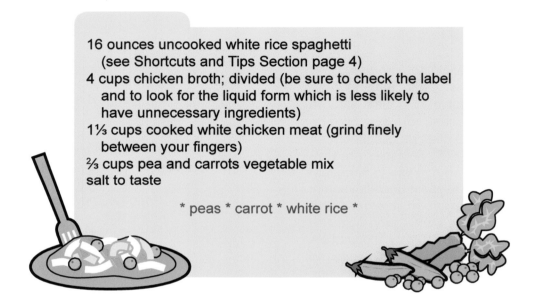

16 ounces uncooked white rice spaghetti
   (see Shortcuts and Tips Section page 4)
4 cups chicken broth; divided (be sure to check the label
   and to look for the liquid form which is less likely to
   have unnecessary ingredients)
1⅓ cups cooked white chicken meat (grind finely
   between your fingers)
⅔ cups pea and carrots vegetable mix
salt to taste

* peas * carrot * white rice *

Bring 3 cups of water to a boil in a pot. Add 2 cups of chicken broth and white rice spaghetti to pot. Stir regularly to mix. When the majority of liquid simmers away, remove spaghetti and rinse quickly with cold water in a colander to clean off any residues that may have formed (much of the chicken broth flavor will be retained in the noodle). Clean pot briefly as well to remove any residue. Add back spaghetti and an additional 2 cups of chicken broth to pot and bring to a simmer. Add peas and carrots and chicken. Simmer and continue to mix regularly. Add salt to taste. When broth has simmered away, remove from heat.

This dish can be served as directed above or you can reserve a Tablespoon or two of broth to add back before serving.

Kid's Shepherd Pie

Meat, vegetables and gravy are mixed into mashed potatoes and then placed into individual bowls. This is then topped with seasoned French fries and baked. This would be a great dish to use homemade mashed or smashed potatoes (see recipe on page 35) as well. Serve with ketchup on the side.

Mashed Potato Base

2 cups instant mashed potato flakes
2 Tablespoons margarine or
   vegetable shortening
¾ cup water (boiling)
⅓ cup vegetable, beef or chicken broth
½ cup cooked vegetables (peas,
   carrots, green beans, corn, broccoli)
salt to taste

Meat and Gravy

¾ cups of uncooked ground beef
2 cups of water
8 Tablespoons instant mashed
   potato flakes
8 Tablespoons vegetable
   shortening or margarine
2 cups vegetable, beef or chicken
   broth
1 ⅓ teaspoon garlic powder
3 Tablespoons balsamic vinegar

Topping

Frozen French fries
½ teaspoon paprika
½ teaspoon onion powder
salt to taste
pepper to taste

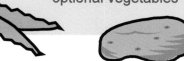

* optional vegetables * potato*

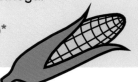 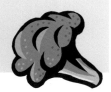

Preheat oven to 375°F.
Prepare Mashed Potato Base. Mix instant potato flakes, margarine, water (boiling) and broth. Add vegetables and salt to taste.
Prepare Meat and Gravy. Place uncooked beef and 2 cups of water in a pan and cook beef over medium heat. You may add additional water if necessary to ensure meat is thoroughly cooked. When there is approximately ¼ cup of liquid remaining at bottom of pan and meat is entirely cooked, remove from heat. Spoon beef out and mix into mashed potato base, leaving liquid behind in pan which will be used to form gravy. To prepare the gravy, add 8 Tablespoons of instant mashed potato flakes, 8 Tablespoons shortening, 2 cups of broth, garlic powder and the balsamic vinegar to the pan containing the beef liquid. Cook over medium heat until thickened and gravy forms.
Spoon a few Tablespoons gravy into small oven safe bowls. Place mashed potato base containing cooked beef on top so that it is now ½ way to ⅔ way up the side of the bowl. Add additional spoons of gravy to top. Cover with French fries and sprinkle with seasonings. Bake for 15 to 20 minutes or until French fries brown nicely.

Mexican Chicken Casserole

This dish meets all your families Mexican cravings. It is also great dish for leftovers.

2 medium sized boneless skinless chicken breasts,
   cooked and chopped into small cubes
3 Tablespoons corn starch
½ cup water
2 cups chicken broth
1 cup rice milk
¾ teaspoon salt
¾ teaspoon paprika
½ teaspoon onion flakes
¼ teaspoon cumin
¼ teaspoon garlic powder
1 cup diced tomatoes plus juice from the can
1 pinch chili powder (optional)
1 cup black beans (drained and rinsed)
½ cup corn
pepper to taste
10 corn tortillas, torn into pieces

* tomato * black beans * corn *

Cook chicken thoroughly by boiling first in water. I like to cut slices in the chicken to help to speed up the cooking and ensure it cooks completely. When cooked set aside. Cut into cubes when cooled.

Preheat oven to 400°F. Place corn starch and all liquid ingredients into a large pot. Stir thoroughly. Add seasonings and salt. Bring to a boil, and let simmer until it starts to get hot and thickens very slightly (some starch may congeal but just keep stirring until it starts to thicken). Once thickened slightly, remove from heat and add chicken, tomatoes, beans, and corn. Stir well. Add the tortilla pieces and stir again. Place into an 8x8 or 9x9 inch baking dish. Bake for 20 to 25 minutes.

Fried Chicken and
Smashed Red Potatoes (with gravy)

Small chicken wing drumsticks are used to ensure they are cooked thoroughly. If you would like to use large drumsticks, more oil and frying time will be required.

Fried Chicken

1 pound chicken wing drumettes
1 cup rice milk
1 cup whole grain brown rice flour
2½ teaspoons paprika
2½ teaspoons oregano
2 teaspoons salt
1 teaspoon garlic powder
¾ teaspoon ginger (not heaping)
canola oil for frying

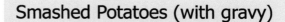

* potato * whole grain brown rice *

Add all dry ingredients to a bowl and mix well. Add rice milk to a separate bowl. Pour oil into a pan so that it is ¼ inch deep and begin heating over medium heat. Dip chicken in rice milk and then flour mixture and place in frying pan. Turn often until chicken is browned on all sides (approximately 7 to 10 minutes) and is thoroughly cooked on the inside. Remove from heat and drain on paper towel.

Smashed Potatoes (with gravy)

8 red potatoes
8 Tablespoons vegetable shortening or
    margarine
8 Tablespoons Instant Mashed Potato
    Flakes
2 cups chicken broth
1 ⅓ teaspoon garlic powder
salt to taste

Bring potatoes to a boil in water and then turn down to medium heat and allow to cook for 20 minutes. Remove and allow to cool. Cut into quarters and place in a bowl and set aside.
To make gravy, heat vegetable shortening or margarine over medium heat. Add potato flakes and mix well. Add chicken broth. Bring to a simmer and continue to cook until most of the liquid has boiled away and sauce thickens. Remove from heat. Add garlic powder and salt to taste.
Using a fork or potato smasher, mash potatoes slightly. Pour in gravy and mix well.

No Noodle Lasagna

You won't miss noodles in this dish because it has so much depth. Breaded zucchini is added to breaded chicken cutlet with a great tomato sauce base. Try some of the additional options to add even more dimension. The combined flavors are great. You can serve with white rice noodles, rice, sliced potatoes or French fries on the side.

Three breaded cooked chicken cutlets (page 30)
    or 12 cooked Chicken Nuggets (page 22)
2 cups tomato juice
1 cup cooked carrot puree
1 cup well cooked broccoli florets
2 zucchinis with skins removed, sliced lengthwise
1 cup rice milk
½ cup whole grain brown rice flour
¾ teaspoon salt
2½ Tablespoons apple cider vinegar
salt to taste
canola oil for frying

* zucchini * carrot * tomato * broccoli *
whole grain brown rice *

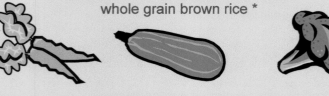

Additional Options:

Ground beef added to tomato broccoli sauce

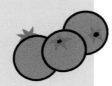

    Eggplant layers

    Turkey sausage added to
       tomato broccoli sauce

    Bacon layers

Prepare breaded chicken cutlets or nuggets and then preheat oven to 375°F. Prepare tomato broccoli sauce. Add tomato juice, carrot puree and broccoli to pan and cook over medium heat until slightly thickened. Remove from heat. Prepare zucchini. Mix brown rice flour and ¾ teaspoon of salt in a bowl. Mix well. Dip zucchini in rice milk and place in rice flour mixture to coat. Add canola oil to pan so that it is approximately a ¼ inch deep. Bring up to medium to high heat. Add zucchini and fry until both sides are slightly browned (a few minutes). Remove from heat and place on paper towels to drain and then on a dish. Pour cider vinegar over zucchinis.

In an oven safe casserole dish, add a layer of tomato sauce, a layer of zucchini, a second layer of tomato sauce, and on top of this place breaded chicken (use all breaded chicken in this layer). Add a strip of tomato sauce down the middle of the chicken so it just covers ⅓ of the chicken. Add the second layer of zucchini on top and pour over a third layer of sauce. Make sure there is sufficient room on top of the casserole dish that is empty to prevent bubbling over of sauce. Place in oven and bake for 15 to 20 minutes. Allow to cool somewhat before serving.

Chewy Chocolate Brownies

Just like the brownies you grew up on. Make sure to use the carrot puree, do not replace with another egg replacer as you will be so surprised how well it works with chocolate. Also, the trick to chewy brownies is to place the brownie pan in a bath of freezing cold water immediately when removed from the oven. Cooling quickly locks chewiness in the center. I also use a cupcake pan as this recipe is prone to the brownies sinking if a large pan is used.

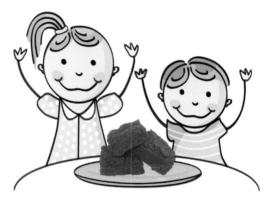

1 cup salt free margarine or vegetable shortening
   (measure prior to melting)
1 cup cocoa
1½ cup whole grain brown rice flour
2 cups white sugar
1 cup corn starch
3 Tablespoons of arrowroot
½ teaspoon salt
½ teaspoon baking powder (recipe page 4)
1 cup cooked carrot puree
Foil cupcake liners (prevents the brownies from sinking)

* carrot * whole grain brown rice *

Preheat oven to 375°F. Melt shortening in a pan over medium heat. Remove from heat and add cocoa. Stir until smooth. Mix all dry ingredients in a bowl. Add the shortening and cocoa mixture. Batter will be the consistency of icing. Mix well. Place foil liners in cupcake wells. Fill wells ¾ of the way full with batter. I like to add an extra dollop of batter to the center portion of each well as an extra preventative against sinking in the middle. Place in oven and cook for 25 minutes on the middle rack.

Remove and immediately place pan into a cold bath (I use my sink and create a shallow cold water bath – place pan in carefully and make sure that no water seeps into brownie pan). Allow brownies to cool in water bath and then remove.

Brownies can be left at room temperature in a ziplock bag (they will be even chewier the next day) or they can be stored long term in the freezer.

Tip

If the brownies are not chewy enough it may be because of the cocoa brand you are using. I have tried this with different cocoa brands and depending on the brand you may need to add more carrot puree to the recipe to achieve chewiness.

Unbelievably Fast Light and Fruity Muffins

Such fun - light, fluffy and moist muffins that you can add any of your favorite fruit to and ready in 5 minutes as they are cooked in the microwave! You pour, cook and <u>serve</u> them in a microwavable cup or I prefer a small deep bowl. Makes 2 muffin bowls.

¼ cup whole grain brown rice flour
¼ cup plus 1 Tablespoon corn starch (note you cannot replace the corn
    starch with tapioca starch in this recipe)
1 teaspoon baking powder (recipe page 4)
1½ teaspoons sugar
1½ Tablespoons applesauce
2½ Tablespoons maple syrup
2½ Tablespoons of canola oil
¼ cup plus 1 Tablespoon rice milk
¼ cup favorite fruit (if necessary chop into small pieces)

* apple * favorite fruit (optional) * whole grain brown rice *

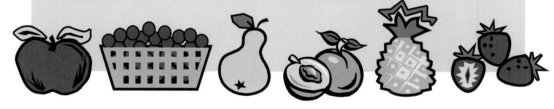

Mix all dry ingredients well. Add remaining ingredients and mix well again. Batter will be very thin which is important to making muffins moist. Pour ½ cup of batter into a microwave safe cup or small bowl. Microwave times will vary depending on your microwave but try starting at 45 seconds on HIGH. Muffin should appear "set" (not wet to touch) and should appear light and fluffy. If the muffin is not ready, try microwaving and testing at 10 second intervals until fully cooked. Allow the muffin to cool in the bowl. It is also important to allow the bowl to cool as the muffin will be seved in the bowl. Once this is done, serve muffin immediately. Muffin will dry out quickly if allowed to sit around too long.

38

Chocolate Ice Cream

Many rice milk ice creams contain soy. You will see this is absolutely not necessary though you will need to invest in a small ice cream maker, which is absolutely worth it! You may be required to modify the recipe below according to your manufacturer's instructions.

2 cups rice milk; divided
¼ cup sugar
½ cup cocoa
3 teaspoons corn starch

Add corn starch to 3 Tablespoons of rice milk. Mix until smooth. Heat remaining rice milk in a pan. Just prior to boiling, remove the rice milk from heat and add corn starch: rice milk mixture to pan. Place back on stove top over low heat, stirring constantly until mixture thickens (will take minutes). The corn starch may start to gel, just continue stirring well until the mixture thickens. Remove from heat and add sugar. Mix well. Pour in a bowl and add chocolate. Stir until melted. Place in refrigerator (not freezer) overnight. Follow ice cream makers specific directions.

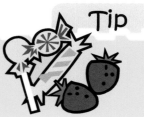

Tip

Follow manufacturer instructions and try adding your child's favorite fruit or crushed candy.

Plain, Chocolate or Vanilla Icing

½ cup Tablespoons vegetable
 shortening
¼ cup powdered sugar
¼ cup cocoa (optional)
 or 1 Tablespoon vanilla extract
 (optional)

Plain:
Mix shortening and sugar well in a bowl.

Chocolate:
Melt shortening in a pan over medium heat. Remove from heat. Stir in cocoa powder and mix well. Place in a covered bowl in the refrigerator and allow to solidify (about 30 minutes). Add powdered sugar and mix well again.

Vanilla:
Mix shortening and vanilla extract in a bowl. Add powdered sugar and mix well again.

Chocolate Cake or Cupcakes

Boiling the rice milk is important as it removes graininess of the brown rice flour. As with the brownies, be sure to use the cooked carrot puree, do not replace as it is a wonderful egg replacer with chocolate desserts. Serve with vanilla or chocolate icing. Makes one 9 inch square cake or 8 to 10 cupcakes.

1 cup whole grain brown rice flour
⅓ cup instant mashed potato flakes
2½ Tablespoons tapioca starch
½ cup cocoa
1 cup sugar
⅓ teaspoon salt
2 teaspoons baking powder (recipe page 4)
5 Tablespoons canola oil
3 Tablespoons cooked carrot puree
1 teaspoon vanilla extract (optional)
1 cup rice milk (boil just before adding)

* carrot * potato * whole grain brown rice *

Preheat oven to 350°F. Mix all dry ingredients well. Add all remaining ingredients *except* rice milk and mix well again. Boil rice milk in a pan (do not allow much to evaporate) and add immediately to mixture. Stir well and quickly to make sure everything is mixed well and evenly dispersed. Note batter will be very thin.

Pour into a 9 inch square pan or fill cupcake pan almost full (cupcakes will not rise much). Bake cake for 30 to 40 minutes and cupcakes 15 to 20 minutes or until a toothpick comes out clean.

Hot Chocolate

This is so simple for a cold day. Try adding the optional carrot puree to thicken. They will never know it's in there and as I've said in other dessert recipes, it is amazing paired with chocolate.

2⅓ cups water
¼ cup sugar
3 Tablespoons cocoa
¼ cup cooked carrot puree (optional)

* carrot (optional) *

Mix all ingredients in a pan. Mix well and cook over medium heat until slightly thickened. Allow to cool to an appropriate temperature prior to drinking.

Chocolate Pudding

You will not miss anything in this authentic chocolate pudding recipe. You'll wonder why everyone doesn't make it this simple! Makes 4 small bowls.

4 cups rice milk; divided
½ cup sugar
5 Tablespoons cocoa
6 teaspoons corn starch

* whole grain brown rice *

Add corn starch to 6 Tablespoons of rice milk. Mix until smooth. Heat remaining rice milk in a pan. Just prior to boiling, remove the rice milk from heat and add corn starch:rice milk mixture to pan. Place back on stove top over low to medium heat, stirring constantly until mixture thickens (will take at least 5 minutes and possibly a few minutes longer). If the mixture begins to gel, continue stirring hard while heating until the mixture has thickened to a pudding consistency. Remove from heat and add sugar. Pour in a bowl and add chocolate. Stir until melted. Place in refrigerator. Pudding will be ready within a couple of hours!

Peach Crumble

I remember having my first fruit crumble and thinking this is now my favorite dessert. It is so easy to make and works great with white rice flour. Makes 4 small individual bowls.

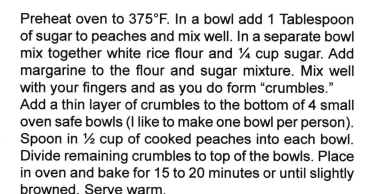

2 cups cooked peaches
1 Tablespoon sugar
⅔ cup white rice flour
¼ cup sugar
6 Tablespoons margarine
    or vegetable shortening
salt to taste (if using vegetable shortening
    you may require additional salt to crumble)

* peaches * white rice *

Preheat oven to 375°F. In a bowl add 1 Tablespoon of sugar to peaches and mix well. In a separate bowl mix together white rice flour and ¼ cup sugar. Add margarine to the flour and sugar mixture. Mix well with your fingers and as you do form "crumbles."
Add a thin layer of crumbles to the bottom of 4 small oven safe bowls (I like to make one bowl per person). Spoon in ½ cup of cooked peaches into each bowl. Divide remaining crumbles to top of the bowls. Place in oven and bake for 15 to 20 minutes or until slightly browned. Serve warm.

Crispy Rice Cereal Treats

You've all had these so no explanation necessary! Make sure rice cereal, gelatin and vanilla are gluten free. Makes enough bars to fill a 13 X 9 inch casserole dish. This is a great place to add raisins or dried cranberries as well.

2 packages unflavored gelatin
½ cup ice cold water
1 cup
⅔ cup corn syrup
¼ cup confectioners sugar
¼ cup instant potato flakes
1½ Tablespoons salt free margarine or vegetable shortening
7 cups rice cereal
1 teaspoon vanilla extract (optional)
½ cup chocolate (optional)
1 cup raisins or dried cranberries (optional)

* raisins or cranberries (optional) * whole grain brown rice *

In a large pot, add water and bring to a boil. Add sugar and corn syrup and continue heating. Allow mixture to bubble and thicken but continue stirring, approximately 3 to 5 minutes. Remove from heat and add shortening. If you are adding vanilla or chocolate add here and mix until dissolved. Add confectioner's sugar and potato flakes. Mix until dissolved. Immediately stir in rice cereal working quickly to coat cereal. Quickly transfer to an appropriate size casserole dish and allow to cool at room temperature. Cut individual squares and cover tightly with saran wrap to prevent drying out.

Carrot or Zucchini Cupcakes

This is a jam packed nutritious cupcake with an option of adding chocolate. Makes 10 to 12 cupcakes.

1⅓ cup plus 2½ Tablespoons whole grain brown rice flour
½ cup plus 2½ Tablespoons instant potato flakes
⅓ cup plus 2 Tablespoons tapioca starch
½ teaspoon salt
2 teaspoons baking powder (recipe page 4)
1⅓ cups granulated sugar
2 teaspoons ground cinnamon
1½ cup raisins (optional)
2 cups peeled and shredded carrots or zucchini
1 cup oil
⅓ cup apple sauce
2 teaspoons vanilla extract (optional)
¾ cup rice milk

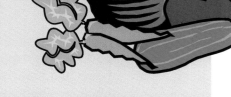

* apple * raisins (optional) * carrot or zucchini * potato * whole grain brown rice *

Preheat oven to 375°F. Mix all dry ingredients well. Bring rice milk to a quick boil in a pan over medium to high heat. Do not allow rice milk to evaporate. Add boiled rice milk directly to flour and stir quickly to dissolve flour mixture. Add all remaining ingredients. Mix well. Fill cupcake wells ¾ of the way full (cupcakes will rise only slightly while cooking). Bake for 20 to 25 minutes or until a fork or toothpick comes out clean.

Tip

Add ½ cup of cocoa powder to this recipe to make chocolate carrot or zucchini cupcakes.

Crunchy Toffee

This is a recipe for older children. You make toffee by boiling sugar at a high temperature but you have to be careful not to let it burn. In my method you do not require a candy thermometer.

¼ vegetable shortening or margarine
2 cups sugar
4 Tablespoons water
¼ teaspoon salt (only if vegetable shortening or a
   salt free margarine is used)
Dairy, Soy, Gluten, Wheat free Chocolate chips
   (optional)

Have a jelly roll pan on hand. Melt margarine or shortening in a pan over low heat. Add sugar. If you are adding salt, add it here. Raise temperature to medium heat, continuously mix with a whisk until sugar has melted and is no longer granular (sugar will *melt* but expect it to remain a separate suspension from the oil). Note once the sugar is no longer granular and has melted you will be looking for sugar to turn to a light brown caramel color (though sugar will continue to be a separate suspension from the oil). Once the light caramel color is achieved, remove IMMEDIATELY from heat or else it will burn quickly. This light caramel color is key to preventing burning and once you see it remove pan from heat.

Quickly pour contents into pan. You will see the oil will separate to the top and the caramel color melted sugar will be on the bottom of the pan. Let sit 2 minutes and then place pan under running faucet with COLD water to wash away oil at the top. Do not worry about washing away the bottom toffee portion in this step. While the water is washing away the top oil the cold water will actually help to solidify the toffee. Once this occurs, use a paper towel to dry any remaining water that is on top of the toffee. You can place in a freezer for a few minutes to help harden as well. If you would like to add chocolate to top, melt chocolate chips and pour on top of toffee and place back in freezer until solidified.

Tips

#1 – toffee can be chopped in the blender and makes a great crunchy topping on the icing of cakes as well as an ice cream addition.

#2 - you can purchase dairy, soy and gluten free chocolate chips online.

Chocolate Chip Cookies

This is the one additional dessert that may require buying a chocolate bar or chips that are dairy, soy and gluten free. They are available and can be purchased online. Alternatively, this is a great cookie in itself without any chocolate chips or chunks. Makes approximately 8 cookies.

½ cup melted margarine or vegetable shortening
(measure after melting is important for this recipe)
1 cup whole grain brown rice flour
1 cup powdered sugar
4 Tablespoons corn starch
dairy, soy and gluten free chocolate chips or bar cut
into small chunks

* whole grain brown rice *

Mix whole grain brown rice flour and powdered sugar in a bowl. Melt margarine or shortening in a pan until just boiling. Measure melted margarine or shortening ½ cup exactly. Add melted margarine or shortening to bowl and mix quickly and well with rice flour and sugar. Dough will be more crumbly than wet.

Preheat oven to 375°F. With your hands take a piece of dough and form into a small ball. Place ball on the cookie sheet and pat down with your hand to form the shape of a cookie working on the cookie sheet (it will end up mound shaped and will be somewhat higher in the middle portion of the cookie). Repeat this with remaining dough. Given the crumbly nature of the dough, you may have some extra crumbly pieces at the end that can not form into a ball but that is okay.

Push several chocolate chips or small chocolate chunks onto the tops of cookie. They only need to be slightly pushed in. If the dough starts to crack or crumble a bit, just work to reform cookie. Bake for 12 to 15 minutes or until nicely browned. Must allow to cool at room temperature before removing with a spatula.

CPSIA information can be obtained
at www.ICGtesting.com
Printed in the USA
LVIC05n0252130514
385509LV00004B/11

9 780984 505708